I0101969

TRAIN THE TRAINER
WHAT PERSONAL TRAINERS MUST KNOW TO SUCCEED AS A PHYSICAL FITNESS EXPERT

BY

TOM TYPINSKI

TRAIN THE TRAINER

Copyright © 2014 Tom Typinski

ISBN:

978-0-9907776-2-5
978-0-9907776

Published by TypinInc

Warren, Michigan

I dedicate this book to the clients I've had the pleasure of working with throughout the years. Without you, I would not have had the rewards of helping families, friends and relatives to grow in fitness. I am still learning.

Thank you

Train The Trainer

TRAIN THE TRAINER

INDEX

INTRODUCTION

WHY TRAINERS ARE IMPORTANT

The best athletes in the world have coaches, trainers, regimens and required exercises to keep them at their optimum condition. Why shouldn't the average athlete? How many everyday skiers, golfers, tennis players, etc., have training built into their off season or pre-season practices?

ANSWER: Those who care to improve.

The gym is more than grunts and groans, throwing weight around or moving endlessly on stationary machines. 80% of the people enrolled in gyms are these automatons who continually go, day after day, week to week, logging in gym hours without ever making positive changes in their bodies.

A trainer will take what you're already doing and add intensity, focus, goals and safety to the client's workout regimens, while taking them to new levels of capability and comprehension. A good trainer will bring out the best in a client. A great trainer will take the client to levels they'd never dreamed possible.

A trainer will show how muscles should work throughout a movement, how they connect, accommodate and support the body parts, and how to get the most out of each particular exercise in a safe fashion, without over or under training.

A trainer will also be a companion on this road to improvement; often garnering great friendships and connections. Not every trainer aspires to, nor is capable of this, yet the best do it effortlessly.

WHY TRAINERS NEED TO READ THIS BOOK

This occupation has taken an inconsistent path toward wellness and fitness. Many trainers are in it for the wrong reasons. It is not all that glamorous, it pays well if you work your butt off, like any other field; but it's not easy, it's not consistent and it's become flooded with too many sub-par practitioners.

Just because you've dieted for a show, or won a contest, or helped your girlfriend lose 10 pounds, doesn't make you a trainer.

Neither does reading a textbook, doing online tests, jumping through the numerous hoops that million dollar, multi level clubs make you go through to wear their brand; or even owning your own gym.

A real trainer has worked for years in various disciplines and sports, read exhaustingly on the research that so often changes; but most importantly, has done years of exercise and can demonstrate a multitude of approaches to honestly assist others in achieving their goals. And they are PASSIONATE.

I often say I will help others even if they don't ask for it; meaning, I will stop someone from doing a bad movement, or show them proper or alternative techniques to get the most out of what they are attempting to do, in a friendly, convincing manner. I help even if I don't have to. I LOVE helping others.

Trainers have become sloppy and lazy, with no real rhyme or reason for their tactics other than having a gullible someone to follow their advice. It's time to earn your respectable place in a very important business. Our work is paramount. Live up to the calling.

CHAPTER 1

MEETING THE CUSTOMER

"It starts with a handshake and hello"

Your focus must be on helping people and supporting their success. You will provide the knowledge, steps and tools to assist them. They can hold you accountable as long as you can hold them accountable; it has to be a clearly understood, mutual proposition.

If they are not the type of client you enjoy working with, or if their goals are too far out of reach for either of you to believe, let them know immediately and part as friends.

The first meeting with a prospective client must remain centered on them. Use the old adage of having two ears and one mouth, to listen twice as much as you talk. They really don't care about you, your cleverness, your victories, your past clients, or your own personal workouts. They care about:

1. What you are going to do for them
2. How long it will take
3. How realistically feasible is it
4. How much it will cost
5. When can they start working out

You must be a gentleman or gentle woman; no swearing, cursing, gossip, slurred words, short, curt or smart-ass responses, and no "know it all" attitudes. They are there to invest time and money in themselves and their welfare must be foremost on their minds, from "hello' to "goodbye." You must earn their trust before attempting friendship, and don't expect friendship. Answer questions with clear, understandable responses. Don't try to impress with scientific jargon or long-winded explanations on the philosophy of exercise. This is still their time, and unnecessary ramblings will give them pause in choosing you. Be succinct, polite, to the point and thorough.

If they came to you as a referral, do not compare them to their friend. You must talk highly of that other person so they are assured you will positively reflect them back to the referral. You are an employee, not a friend. Bad language, bad attitude, bad information will only make you look - you guessed it - bad.

You have a great responsibility and a privilege to live up to working with them. You need to be gracious, not arrogant. They *can* live without you, and will if you wrong them.

You must be realistic in the goals they propose for themselves, giving an honest timeline of what you will do, in order to get them to where they want to be.

Be definitive in what they can expect, good and bad. Explain that the new muscle they will be building comes from beneath the fat which lays on top, from the bone outward; and both fat and muscle will be reversed as long as they are persistent in training, diet, sleep and intensity of focus. But both fat and muscle will be present as they're building new muscle cells and this may cause a "thicker" appearance.

The more they adhere the to training and advice, the sooner they will attain the cuts and definition they had only before dreamed of. The more they refuse to stick to the prescribed regimen, the longer the journey to improvement.

As a trainer, you have two, maybe three hours per week to which they're accountable. You cannot babysit their entire lifestyle and they must know that you are there to make them "work" during their workouts, toward your mutual goal of improving their health, fitness, and life.

Give them a guided timeline to which they can trust you to be there for them, and they to be there for you. Give them access to as much contact information as necessary; phone, email, text, but make clear that this information is for business purposes only, in both directions.

Keep professional distance and they will respect that more than too constant "check ins" over their personal lives. Don't allow them to stalk you as well, over any trivial thing that comes up. Keep the relationships professional, and in the gym only.

Make sure they understand your strengths as a trainer. Do not lead them to believe you can do something for them if you don't know how to achieve what they're asking for. Do not fake a specialization if you only want their money, you will be discovered and lose trust.

Show them around the facility. Tell them the pertinent facts about gym hours, classes offered, rates and availability. Make them commit to a schedule that is workable for both of you if they decide to accept your training.

This initial meeting with the customer can make or break a successful sale and perhaps a long run with them as a client. You must listen and understand where they are coming from, as much as where they want to go toward their goals.

Listening cannot be stressed enough. If they ultimately would like to compete as a physique athlete, do not tell them you know what it takes if you do not really know what it takes. Tell them you can help them to a certain point, and that you will direct them to someone who specializes in the finishing portions of competition, with posing, suit selection, tanning, etc.

The same goes for nutrition. If it's general information they seek, you should be able to provide adequate guidelines to help them understand and enforce good diet habits.

But if they have certain conditions like diabetes, Crohn's or fibromyalgia; or physical deformities which limit their ability, you must know when to say no if these aren't things in your bag of expertise. It raises your credibility instead of lowering it.

BRING IT BACK TO THEM

At the end of this initial consultation, evaluate what you've heard and develop a plan. If they have a particular sport they participate in, even on the most basic, recreational level, tell them how your training can add to their enjoyment and participation in their sport of choice.

All runners, golfers, skiers and weekend athletes have room to grow stronger, faster, more agile, more flexible and more able to participate in their sport.

Sell them on something they already enjoy and tell them how you can enhance their experiences. Even bowlers can enjoy the attributes found in an exercise program.

Repetitive stress injuries are caused by weaknesses in the surrounding structures and accommodating muscles, not just the weakened joint. Enhanced circulation, respiration and flexibility will add comfort as well as confidence to the average athlete's game.

As a trainer, you should have a deep well of programs to fit any person's goals. As long as the benefits are clearly explained, the sale is as close as walking them through the first workout.

CHAPTER 2

DESIGNING WORKOUTS

"A TRAINER CAN EITHER INCREASE INTENSITY OR DURATION"

The greatest benefits are gathered in a reasonable amount of time when an optimum level of energy can be sustained. When the energy falls off, the workout drops, intensity wavers, injuries are possible.

By executing the wrong movement, or an inadequate movement, you are rehearsing your muscle and nervous system and promoting inadequate exercise to the muscle group.

A trainer's responsibility is to recognize when the exercise turns from beneficial to detrimental. A trainer must also be able to recognize when more can be accomplished. Inadequate stimulation is just as bad as too much.

The trainer must pay full attention to his trainees. It's up to the trainer to make sure each rep is extended through the greatest range of motion to benefit the client toward their goals. Why waste time? Why waste a rep? Your client's time is valuable. Give them the best of what you have and move on.

The trainer must vigilantly monitor their prospects' progress. They must push their people as far as anything they would ever put themselves through. A trainer should also not expect more of their people than they themselves would or could do - at least on a personal training level.

Your dedication to continuous training has a mentoring effect, which you can enhance by offering help and tuition and in return, benefitting again by learning as you're teaching. If you know something well enough to teach someone else, you know it well.

There is obviously not a "one size fits all" workout. But there are your philosophies and beliefs and trials and accomplishments. You must never say you have "the way." But, you must always have "a way." You must have a formula, a routine, a discipline that is easy to understand and enforce.

They want to be dependent on you and don't want to be responsible for a workout when you're not around. You must work to change that. You must help and insist they get to the "turn the corner" moment when exercise will become second nature and they'll look forward to it.

Work on a few basic things, day to day, week to week, for the first month. Depending on their level of fitness and willingness to learn, they will be challenged to greater and greater workouts. Not all of them needs to be grueling, but you must have the capacity to push them and the knowledge to know when to back off.

Make the set and rep schemes easy enough to follow so they can anticipate what's coming. This builds confidence and self-esteem. The more you empower them, the more they will ask for and the more they will appreciate what you've given them.

If you're teaching consistency and discipline, than your instructions must carry the same degree of consistency. If you are instilling a routine of "3 of these…and a few of those…then over here for a couple of this…." you are not training them, you are distracting them from doing real work.

A house does not get built when you put "a brick on one side, then two on another, then another over here…" That trendy, circuit type workout has been around for ages. It is still trying to catch on, in numerous incarnations. It's bullshit. It's a trainer winging it. They will run as fast as they can for a substitute. Challenge them to keep raising the stakes.

Weight training will always, ALWAYS, be the go-to method for fitness. Does your favorite Pro Football team do Bosu or Bench Press? Do sprinters do Squats or Pilates? Do hockey players Zumba? No. No. And no! Some may supplement with other disciplines, but every professional athlete uses weights in training for their sport.

If you know the basics and can teach them proficiently, it is like teaching a child to ride a bike. The client will be forever grateful, and you can be happy knowing you've taught others something as vital and satisfying as reading and writing. The fundamental skills in the weight room are as important as any other sport's fundamentals.

PRACTICE WHAT YOU PREACH

The best way to design a workout is to go with something that worked for you in the past. You can relate to the intensity, the weight, the combinations of movements and how to best pace them through it. You should not offer workouts in combinations of movements, rep ranges or apparatus that you are not familiar with yourself.

"Tried and true," need not be boring and pedantic. Variety can be included in the types of movements and apparatus used, as long as correct demonstration of technique is understood and enforced.

WORKING AROUND INJURIES

No matter what goals the client my initially come in with, the primary goal for all clients is "NO WEAK LINKS."

The body is a chain of muscles and tendons, joints and axes. Like a chain, it is only as strong as its weakest link. If a shoulder, knee or back are impaired, the initial remedy should come in strengthening those aspects of the body before attempting to increase or decrease size, strength, or weight, in any other part of the body.

If, as a trainer, you ignore these weaknesses and push through to appease the client or yourself, you are doing a disservice to the client, compromising their health, and possibly making them weaker and further injured in the long run.

Many men favor training the arms and chest, over and over, while skipping abs or legs or any other bodypart. Your job is to take them places they will not go alone. Don't pretend the abdominal and back muscles are not there, despite being hidden by layers of fat. That is all the more reason to work them and strengthen them in support of the core.

When women come and only expect to work their legs or butt, without doing the basic exercises to strengthen the overall structure of the body; you must ensure that working the body, from every angle, will allow their butt and legs to shape faster and easier by adding muscle to the entire body.

"No weak links" means toes to earlobes, mind to muscles, stronger in every aspect, on every plane of movement. You must be the motivator and instigator, with a set plan and the back-up reasoning for its need.

Office workers have multiple neck, shoulder and back weaknesses. Their jobs force them down and forward for days in a row, months on end. You must open the chest, shoulders, collarbones and back "like a swan dive" to help them pull all that office/driving/ desk tension out of their bodies and open them up.

If they have a limitation, you must have two remedies to work around it. Your job is to alleviate those limitations and show them what's possible, despite their aches, with exercises utilizing their healthy body groups.

If they are truly injured with cast, crutches or sling, you must make certain their limitations given them by their doctor are not to be exceeded by you. Find remedies in movement and the tools to help assist in their rehabilitation without pandering or dismissing its value. If you are not versed in rehabilitative training, get them to someone who is or turn them away.

They will just as gratefully accept your honesty as they will your help; and if you insist they rest or go to rehab as ordered, they will graciously accept your professionalism and come back to you when able. There is no need to compromise your client nor your reputation by saying you know what to do, when you don't.

A good trainer can read a client's level of pain or lack of range; a great trainer knows how to work around injuries with a knowledge of physiology, anatomy and "drama detector" when the complaints don't ring true. Feedback and attentive focus can heal most commons sprains and pulls. If you are in doubt, change course, or employ a specialized opinion.

AVOID THE TRENDY

Some trainers pride themselves on knowing all the latest tools and tricks to challenge clients. More power to them. The problem is, they give fundamental instruction and often functional assistance, but immeasurable results. People want two primary things:

1. *To notice visible changes in their bodies*

2. *To have others notice visible changes in their bodies*

Leave the grace and posture and fluidity of movement for the ballroom; more than anything, people want to be seen by the pool, on the boat, at the picnic, able to take their shirts off, shamelessly; or to wear limb baring clothes to the summer soiree.

No one cares how long you can balance on one leg doing a twenty pound curl while holding a kettle bell with the opposite foot, resembling a character out of Dr. Seuss! Unless your sport involves acrobatics, you should train and practice with two feet on the ground. One-footed plyometric exercises are great when tuned to a particular sport with individualized attention to technique; but to the common man or woman, you are showing them another thing the cannot do.

Trendy moves with bands and balls are for people who would rather "play" than "work" out. It sometimes looks "cool" or "tough," but just as you are what you eat, you are how you compete. You never hear of "Buns of Bosu", or "Abs of Rubberbands,"; no, you hear "steel" and "iron," not "plastic."

"Cut, Ripped, Shredded, Defined," are synonymous with "Strength." You will never hear of a body built by "TRX Bands." Respect yourself and your client. Don't play with toys.

If they are in shape and it shows, it speaks volumes for the work they're putting in; and guess who the eventual benefactor is? If you make them feel like a putz, guess what they look and feel like, doing it? And guess what their bodies become? Avoid the trends, IRON RULES!

AN EXAMPLE OF "A WAY" TO TRAIN INDIVIDUALS

One approach is to take a basic, compound movement that involves two or more joints, like the Bench Press, and do 4 sets;

- the first being light and incorporating full range of motion
- the second a little heavier, incorporating adjustments
- a third, heavy set which tests balance and strength
- and a fourth, lighter set that brings it all together

Take a second exercise which works the same muscle group from a different plane of movement, or with different apparatus, like an incline or decline bench with dumbbells, and follow the same protocol of sets.

Do a third exercise, this time very specific to the muscle group, like cable flyes or pec deck, and point out the specific feeling involved in the movement. Point out the differences in the levels and note where they need more help and focus.

This can be done with any muscle group; and the trainer can build a whole-body workout to suit the client's needs based on corresponding exercises which stimulate muscle growth from varied angles. It is easy to understand, simple to employ and an effective system that can be built upon, week to week, month to month. For additional workouts see:

http://www.shockandawemuscle.com for an entire book of high-caliber workouts, systems and advanced training methods.

CHAPTER 3
CONFIDENTIALITY

You must respect and defend the people you are working with by keeping all matters private. You may work with doctors, lawyers, therapists, high-powered executives or other influential people and no matter what they disclose to you, you must not repeat it to others; of course, unless it were to harm someone.

This builds trust. If you work in one particular facility, it's guaranteed that others will know each other and word will always get around, and always come back to you, often misinterpreted or misquoted. The communities they belong to do not often include you, and their alliance to them is stronger than it is to you. Honor that, respect that, and assure them that you can be trusted with whatever information they wish to share.

The best course of action to take is to keep all conversations confidential. You may hear of disgruntled spouses or infidelities; you may hear nuances of patients who may know your other clients, or members of a community who hold influence; and their opinions, vented secretly between them and you, are best kept between only you two. They must be held in confidence to protect the speaker as well as the listener.

If you are known in any degree to betray confidences or alliances, you will lose future prospects. If you share discreet and confidential information with peers and colleagues of your club, word will come back to you, and will become your burden whether you were actively involved or not. You are the least common denominator in anyone's food chain. If anyone falls, you will be first.

AVOID THE DRAMA

There is no need to dramatize this information. There may be times when you're privy to someone pouring their heart out and you are the only listener. Be considerate, calm, neutral, consoling and helpful if possible. This is just to preempt if it does occur. You will know how to handle it.

Often, it's more a case of endless stories about their cats or kids or spouses; and as long as you keep them focused on moving through the workouts, you just have to keep nodding as you would to any other conversation you really don't care to hear. That too is part of your job and there is no need to share these events with coworkers or mutual acquaintances.

Clients tell you these things to either get them off their chest, or to alleviate boredom. If you're not capable of carrying your end of a conversation, to introduce wit or wisdom or knowledge to the workout, you are failing at a very important aspect of the socialization skills necessary to make workouts enjoyable while functional.

Yes, you need to be entertaining! You need to keep the atmosphere light and the workouts heavy, metaphorically speaking. But the topics must be centered on them, their interests, concerns, questions, likes and dislikes, not yours.

And never delve into the personal. It may happen and you are unable to stop it, but divert it or snuff it as early as possible. You really can be gracious in refusing information that has nothing to do with you. Be kind and courteous, but never prying. If they want you to know more, they will tell you.

A TRAINER WEARS MANY HATS

A trainer is more than a person who stands by to observe proper form and monitor the correct execution of exercises. A trainer is a marriage counselor, psychologist, dream interpreter, friend, father, family counselor, financial advisor, mentor, subordinate, peer and taskmaster.

A trainer must know when to use discretion in talking about private matters and when to voice his opinion. He must know when to draw the line in accepting invitations and when to ask for insight or contacts if needed.

There is a line of confidentiality a trainer must never cross. He must constantly instill trust and integrity to his clients through his actions, dialogue and written communications.

A client may test your integrity in the early stages, just to see how noble you really are to his privacy. Don't go for it. Stay out of political, religious, sexual or preferential discussions over any matter they may bring up.

You are there to train them. Stay with the workout, nutrition, injury or training session as topic, but do not stray into siding for or against spouses, children, associates or competing companies. That is not your business.

People can turn on you for an opinion. They can hold a grudge for an off-color remark. There are plenty of things to discuss without delving into the personal lives of you or your client. If it's brought up once, it can be brought up again; and that is an unnecessary gateway to open.

Stay professional by staying engaged in the things the client is doing. They did not sign up with you for a "Social

Membership." The sooner they know that, the more they'll respect it.

You are often their closest companion for hours per week, where they begin to feel they can share things with you that no one else will listen to. The key word is "listen". You can encourage the conversation as much as they wish, but again, stay out of your opinions and in neutrality in regards, especially, to their private matters.

DO NOT COMPARE CLIENTS TO CLIENTS

Competition is good, as long as both sides agree to it. Do not get caught in the trap of telling Client A that Client B is capable of so many reps, so much weight, a certain capability; if they want to know how someone else is doing, answer them simply, but do not compare what one can do, especially if the person asking is the one who cannot.

You may think you're pointing out that Client B has more strength even though they may be smaller or older or whatever the case may be; but what Client A hears, is that they are not good enough, not doing enough, not trying as hard. Both clients have certain abilities and the only way you should compare them is to themselves, how they were a month, week, year ago.

Do not point out that the other client should also be doing better, as a way to point out flaws in their training. If it's flawed, you're responsible, as much or more than the client. The same goes for your colleagues who may have different training styles than your own. Negative comments do no one any good.

By keeping your client focused and attentive to the task at hand, will assure that petty dramas will be kept at bay, and confidentiality be understood as a way of doing business.

CHAPTER 4
HOW TO BECOME A GREAT TRAINER

Someone has come to you for expert advice and guidance. The greatest thing you can do for them, and for yourself, is to give them what they ask for; plain and simple.

If confidentiality is the second best secret to acquiring high powered clientele; the first, of course, is being a good trainer. So how do you become a good trainer? There are many, many, different avenues. Some rely on trendiness. Some rely on mixing it up "to make it interesting". Some change it daily, weekly, monthly; while some never change it at all.

I believe in empowering the client with the knowledge necessary for the tools and facilities he has to deal with, in order to make any gym comfortable and native to his knowledge and ability.

As much as people say they like to change, they really like familiarity and the comfortable confidence that comes with knowing what to do when walking into a gym.

Train them to know the basics, to be proficient at push ups, pull ups, squats and lunges. Teach them the weights to use for dumbbell and barbell and other basic movements/apparatus.

Empower them to the point to where they know it enough to share it. Teach them methods and disciplines that are consistent, yet challenging. Continue to watch their execution over range of motion and economy of movement.

They must learn tempo, pace and space in relation to the muscles they're working. They must know why inclines and declines are different. They must know how to breathe efficiently. They must utilize time efficiently.

They learn all of this from you. Too much talk, too much rest, too much wasted time and you are to blame for a bad workout. Help them look forward to workouts. Encourage them to see the differences in their strength, appearance, demeanor, posture, capabilities. Remind them where they were when they started.

By the same token, being too harsh or demanding can backfire as well. You must be in tune to their capabilities by reading facial nuances, respiration, range of motion and force. You must not patronize them if they cannot do something. No one wants to be made a fool, especially by someone they're paying to help them look cool.

The degree to which you practice these disciplines as a trainer, the greater your ability to teach more clients, and therefore, to help the world with your work. This is the same as a music teacher teaching the very most basic aspects of an instrument; you will either hook them or scare them. Hook them.

I AM HERE TO SHOW YOU WHAT YOU CAN DO, NOT WHAT YOU CANNOT

A trainer must be able to do all that he asks of the client, and more. He must be able to walk the talk. Pull ups, push ups, squats, lunges, sit ups, must be demonstrated with good, if not, great form.

You must instill in each person a benchmark of "if I can, so can you." We're talking rep for rep, not pound for pound. It is the execution of the movement, demonstrated with control and form, that will help the client shape the muscle; not the amount of weight. Your demonstration must set the standard.

Weight is earned through proper technique. Too much weight in sloppy form is an exercise in someone's ego. It's an injustice as a trainer and a dangerous proposition for the client. So if you are demonstrating with a lot of weight, make sure the client understands they don't have to use as much; and that you can execute as they are supposed to do, perfectly. There is no shame in dropping weight to correct and improve form.

There are many, many movements and apparatus that a new client cannot do; your job is to encourage and prove to them what they can do, not what they can't.

If they are unsure, the first thing you must pump up is their confidence. You must also respect that "no means no" if it's too much weight, pain, difficulty, etc. Do not patronize or criticize anyone who really does not have the capacity to do the exercises. Do not compare your degree of physical ability against someone else's, despite size or build or age.

You are there to train them with an understanding of how they must be trained. Rarely should you ask them for advice. But don't be reluctant to question them on the effectiveness of a movement.

It is often a good idea to demonstrate the exercises if they are new to the gym. Explain as you go how the movement works a particular muscle group. The greater the understanding you can impart to them, the quicker they will improve and the further they can ascend. Just know when to stop, so as not to inundate them with too much jargon or information. Tell them only what will help them understand.

THINK LIKE A CUSTOMER

If you were getting lessons for any activity, what would you look for and like in the person you're interviewing? Be that person. Think of how they should be groomed and dressed for the occupation. Think of the language, the questions you would ask and the answers you would most like to hear.

If you are already a trainer and desire to go to the next level as a Master Trainer, what would impress you enough to pay for their services. This is how you should be thinking when walking a new prospect through your gym.

But above all these aspects, a trainer must be able to walk the talk. He must be an ideal to which the client can hold themselves. He must demonstrate perfect form if he's asking for it from the customer and he must identify when something is too hard to accomplish. This simply gives him humanity as well as humility.

Your body is your calling card, not your certificates, credentials, resume or trophy's. If you are in great shape, the client has no excuse not to live up to your ideal. If you are sloppy, slovenly, out of shape, moody or downtrodden, you become the client's problem. There is no need to put that on them. You must be exemplary as a fitness expert, on all levels.

If you must fake it to paint a cheerful disposition on your day, do it. If you are a mental or physical wreck, you're in the wrong business of helping people get healthy. There are times when you have to show you too are human; just don't let that demeanor be your daily countenance. You can be tired or troubled, but do your best to give your best and you will always be appreciated, and a great trainer.

CHAPTER 5
RESPECT

Respect is a mutual admiration. It is a way of mutually showing that you respect the client for coming to and choosing you; and you respect the opportunity to assist them in reaching their fitness goals; while they obviously respect you to aid in their tuition.

You build a relationship with potential clients like you would with any other stranger; the only difference is, they've come to you with questions and needs and you must be able to answer them intelligently. Find some common ground by establishing that you understand their concerns and issues.

Keep them at the forefront of your answers with direct eye contact, clear, distinct language, smiles, nods of agreement and pertinent questions that build on solutions to their problem.

Avoid asides which digress from the topic, like mutual friends, similar backgrounds or social media/entertainment topics. It's easy to get lost or off track. It's up to you to keep the conversation focused and relevant to their needs.

Remember, if you are an appointment-filled trainer, you are interviewing them as much as they are interviewing you.

Let them know you understand their goals. Assure them that you have solutions to their issues. Be realistic about their expectations and ground them in checkpoints and guideposts that you will both keep in mind along the way. If both of you are doing what is required, you will reach the goals sooner and adjustments can be made to realign your common direction.

Make their goals, your goals. None of your other clients need to be included in the conversations or comparisons unless they bring it up as a question. They must be treated respectfully as individuals, with their personal strengths and weaknesses.

POSITIVE SELF-TALK

Your language should always be encouraging, never demeaning, even if trying to kid around. They are sensitive about their strength and abilities; and even if they are self - deprecating, steer them into positive feedback about what they are accomplishing.

Self-talk is an important issue that few trainers fail to take into account. When someone continually says "they can't, they won't, they never will..." abolish it immediately. Show them instantly that they "can, have, and will continue" to achieve.

There is no need to take a "Pollyanna Approach" by being sickeningly optimistic. You can obviously point out that they need to work on form, explosiveness, tempo, balance, etc.; but don't be that parent that sees everything their "little angel" does as infallible.

They don't like to be patronized, and as adults who are used to work reviews and complaint departments, they can take positive criticism. Just don't be so over the top that everyone but you can see how fake it sounds.

Respect is showing up on time, being attentive, notifying changes in appointments and alternative time slots. It means being proactive when a weekend injury compromises the planned workout and a different approach is necessary. It simply means treating them as the coworker they are; making it pleasant to be in each other's company for hours per week.

PUT YOUR TOYS AWAY

1. Keep phones, keys, personal belongings and anything else that have nothing to do with the workout, out of sight.
2. Never, ever keep your cell phone out, or use it around clients.
3. Do not eat or drink anything but water in front of the client.
4. After you are done with an apparatus or piece of equipment, put it away.
5. Replace dumbbells and barbells to respect your fellow trainers, and reflect your sense of responsibility to clients.
6. Re-rack your weights so others know you're finished.
7. Talk minimally to other people and kindly explain you are with a client, but will answer their questions as soon as you are available.
8. Clean up your space after yourself, all towels, papers or pieces of clothing; remember, this is your "house."

These are simple guidelines that should be known and practiced, but too many bad trainers, self-centered trainers, or egocentric trainers who think they are above it, fail. This is simple gym etiquette and if you practice it automatically as a trainer, each client will follow suit, respecting the gym floor and each individual using it.

The ultimate respect is to give time and energy only to that individual client for the allotted session. As long as it stays about "them," you will shine.

CHAPTER 6
TRAINING TEAMS

It is always nice to say you contributed to a winning team; but when you hear you made a difference in one person's life, at a critical time in their life, when no one else saw hope or possibility, you cannot measure the rewards it brings.

If your background comes from being an athlete in a particular sport, a great proving ground of what you know can be found in training teams. You can connect the memory of what you wished you knew then, to what you know now, offering a perspective on the physical aspects rather than the fundamentals, principles and strategies of a coach.

You will see the differences and discrepancies of how the young person moves, where their strengths exist and what they lack. It is often very challenging because they are not well established in strength, coordination and control of their bodies like an adult may be. You will see that some are naturals and some really need specific tuition to simply reach the basic level.

As much as it is challenging, it is rewarding. Teaching children their first push ups or pull ups or sit ups, can make a long-term effect on their futures. If you can do it with tact, optimism and a bit of humor you are doing a service, not only to them, but to every team they compete on. You are contributing to the welfare of countless benefactors with your simple gift of guidance.

Getting the worst player on the team to achieve a great play is as crucial as pushing the star to simply raise his statistics. You have a team to work with, but it's still individualized training.

GET DOWN TO IT AND DO IT WITH THEM

The most important thing you can do to win their respect, is to perform the exercises right alongside them. Nothing is as impressive to a young athlete as a grown up who can walk the talk. We've all experienced fat, out of shape, whistle-toting, clipboard-carrying coaches who smell like cigarettes and get winded from walking the width of the gym floor. You are not them.

A team trainer, from middle school to college, little league to pro, must know how to motivate with positive information and programs that benefit the least gifted was well as the most. You must not allow any "weak links" in your chain of command.

You must work on the weakest and encourage the rest of the team to bring them up to speed; because collectively, their strength comes from camaraderie, commitment, and completing the given exercises with expertise and precision all the way through competition. If any one of them don't live up to their role, the whole team suffers. Drive this point home first and your job becomes easier.

If you have kids who just don't want to listen, who cause more trouble and distraction than contribution, give them some sense of authority. Call them out to demonstrate, to stand at the front, to "lead."

If they are already the biggest and strongest and feel above the repetition of exercise drills, incorporate their ability into your demonstrations so they will be looked up to as an example rather than a goof ball. When someone good goofs off, the rest of the team takes that as the example to follow as the "cool thing"; cut that immediately. Give him authority and the rest of the team will follow that "positive" example instead.

The more you instill the spirit of teamwork in training programs, the better the coaches will be able to work the team toward a common goal, without distractions.

TEAM TRAINING APPROACHES

Training teams takes a well-planned approach that is difficult enough for the most gifted, yet flexible enough to accommodate the less capable athletes.

With body-weight exercises for adolescents, and basic compound movements for secondary school competitors and above, you can build great training regimens that are easy to follow and implement into any sports program.

Incorporate all the methods you would for a personal client:
• Plyometrics
• Strength building exercises
• Stretching
• Equal focus on upper and lower body movements
• A calendar that alternates bodyparts and exercises
• Nutrition counseling
• Rest recommendations

In the end, you will find more ways to work with a wider array of personalities and body styles. Children won't hide pain and are more often apt to celebrate capability.

Team training is also a great place to meet parents who too may employ your expertise at a later date . If you show genuine concern for their child, they will be your best testimonials. Give your best, to get the best, always. And never, ever criticize or condemn any one person for a faulty play caused by many.

TEAM TRAINING IS NOT COACHING

Physical training must be done from the perspective of a friend with authority, a teammate, rather than an authority figure. They must understand that you are there to help them, to improve their game individually, with attention and guidance that will help every aspect of their play in every sport.

Let the coach be the one who dictates the whole team morale and goal. You are a personal trainer to the group, and your job is to make sure each and every one of them is capable of understanding and fulfilling their own physical ability.

A coach may make them understand that they have to get set up so the guy who scores is in position, the forward, guard, running back, whatever the set up is for positioning the best players to do what they do best, score.

A trainer must make each teammate rise to their own best efforts, to be stronger, faster, more attentive, responsive, and automatically use their assets to help the team in their given capacity.

What you'll find with teams of young athletes in general and a few in particular, is their willingness to try new methods and their determination to succeed. The outstanding athletes will rise to the top and push themselves without any need for recognition. They do it because they truly love the challenges, of lifting more weight, moving faster, doing better, outperforming their previous best efforts. This is where you, as a trainer, relearn what is possible and perhaps remember what got you here in the first place. Share in their excitement and victories and build on those memories to create lasting impressions toward the good of competitive play.

CHAPTER 7
WHERE TO FIND WORK

Everyone knows someone who needs training. Start with your family, your friends, your neighbors, your community, your old school, church or volunteer center. Tell them to commit to paying a small fee for you to guide them to better health. Set up a program that states specific days, times, locations and goals. Plan to do it with them if necessary, though not everyone will agree to pay to watch you work out.

This is a great first step to see if you can tolerate the discipline required to be the accountable guardian of someone's health. If you find you can't hack the tardiness, unwillingness, excuses and level of personal energy you must spend to keep them motivated, then this is not your line of work. You've just save thousands of hours and dollars studying to be something you are not cut out to be.

Whatever the impression may be of a trainer, it is not glamorous, sexy or lucrative. It is a hard road to earn a degree of success and the respect it takes to be a professional. Start small, get feedback from those who will give honest assessments of your approach and tactics, then take that advice and hone it before attempting to be a Club Trainer.

In order to be a "people person extraordinaire," you must exhibit patience, understanding, tolerance and a creative mind with a good memory. You must know when to be stern and when to be kind. You must also always do things for the client's greatest good. If you cannot do all of this, find another occupation. If you haven't thought about these aspects, think about them; come up with an approach that is unique to you, and try it out.

There are a great number of certification programs available to the aspiring trainer. First, decide on what type of clientele you wish to dedicate a chunk of your life to:

- Do you work well with children?
- Do you favor athletes?
- Do you wish to work with competitive physique athletes?
- Do you enjoy going to and teaching group classes?
- Do you work well with seniors?
- Do you want to focus on rehabilitation, prevention, nutrition or team performance?

These are crucial questions to ask before embarking on a training certification.

Some people think they can take on anybody who asks of their services. Good trainers are adaptable and able to work at many levels. Great trainers, like great doctors, specialize. You will reach higher fees, a steadier calendar of more dependable patrons who are willing and able to pay for extensive training, greater credibility and a higher success rate as a Master Trainer.

But here, results are all that speak on your resume. There is no in between. You are good, or you are not. Word of mouth is the original social media and it still travels faster than lightening. Once you get established in a community, your recommendations will come from existing clients. But it still comes down to results. You can be know as a hard trainer, an easy trainer, or simply, an effective trainer. So, what kind of trainer do you want to be?

CHAPTER 8
CORPORATE WELLNESS/ TRAINING OUTSIDE THE GYM

This specifically refers to trainers involved in helping companies and their employees outside of a gym setting.

With health care in the self-care state it is currently in, it is becoming more important for people to take their health into their own hands. It takes more than screening services set up by hospitals and changes in the cafeteria food offerings; it takes someone to personally come into the corporate setting as an accountability partner and impart information and programs to reach out to employees who may be reluctant to travel to a gym, or not want to take the time to head to a suitable location.

Programs like "Biggest Winner" are easy to begin. They incorporate lifestyle changes rather than just weight loss contests. The one I do has 11 variables which give each employee points per week on a lifestyle habit that is changed for the good; such as smoking cessation, drinking more water, exercising or walking with a spouse or pet, getting more sleep, eating better foods, keeping a food diary, etc.

These changes are all things anyone can do on their own, and in the corporate setting can be gauged competitively between floors, departments, male/female, etc. They are fun to do and incentivized through the company to reward the top 1-3 participants with some type of prize at the end of 4-6 weeks. One prize involved a weekend stay in an upscale hotel for the winner and their spouse, nice prize for changing their lives.

WEEKLY WALKS

Another easy to incorporate program is a walking route, suitable for all body types, no gym attire required other than a pair of tennis shoes.

Starting weekly walks from the workplace can involve pedometers or different courses based on time and/or distance. This gives employees a chance to socialize outside the workplace, get some fresh air, and return to work more alert, in better moods and healthier with minimal effort.

Both these programs are based on a trust. Most adults will easily comply and police each other if there is a prize involved. If they are on the same team, they will watch out for what the other is eating or drinking. There are all kinds of ways to play this.

Weekly weigh ins can be incorporated for willing participants, because those serious about losing or changing habits will be willing to gain that knowledge about themselves.

INFORMATIVE SEMINARS

Follow up can be done with feedback on how the workers feel after attempting a program for 4-6 weeks; or preempted with informational seminars that educate the workforce on exactly what little changes in habit can bring big lifestyle adjustments. Ergonomics in the workplace, proper lifting and moving techniques, even self-defense classes can be brought to the job site to help show the employees that their owner is invested in their health and security.

A trainer can follow up with newsletters, email information or tips, which can lead to personal training sessions at a later time.

CHAPTER 9

REWARDS

So what is so good about being a trainer? What is it that attracts so many people to this line of work? How can people be so arrogant to think they can create programs for strangers that will ultimately change their lives? How many are truly trying to make a difference, help humanity, leave a legacy? How many are just poseurs?

These questions have been answered in previous chapters. Passion? Yes. Knowledge? Yes. Dedication? Yes. but the underlying, driving motive to be a successful trainer must be found in the rewards of helping others.

A trainer has a great responsibility to enrich the lives of those he come in contact. A trainer must love this work so much that they would and do, perform these duties for free. A trainer is a giver. And the rewards are found in the drops of sweat you contribute to the gym floors of the world.

Your influence goes from client to spouse, to family, to friends, to loved ones and continues in a perpetual ripple through posterity. That's a bold statement? Yes.

But if you are doing a good job, your lessons should outlive you. They should resonate through generations and be handed down with the Wisdom of The Ages. If you can't live up to that, if you're simply following footsteps on a floor that someone else has painted rather than blazing your own trail, you're wasting your's and everyone else's time, money and energy.

You all know these trainers. You have worked with them, listened to their meek spiels of memorized textbood information and rote protocols toward fitness without an ounce of originality or creativity. These are the same ones who complain about not having enough clients, money, ideas to sustain a living. They are the ones that you and your clients scratch your heads in wonder of what they're trying to achieve with their haphazard approaches and inconsistent results.

Building bodies is like building anything else of lasting value and significance; it requires plans, detained information, proper tools, supplies and teamwork. If you are ready to help people create new lifestyles, state your claim and carry on.

If you are in it for money, or glory, or ego, get the hell out and leave the work to the ones who truly know and love their craft.

Reward your client with honest assessments on their progress and things you see changing in their physique. They will be able to read your sincerity when it isn't given too often, and when they too can see and realize it.

People always want to know they're doing good, and pleasing you as well; though some secretly don't feel it's about your validation. They still want to hear that you're proud of the work they're doing, and that they are doing things in a right manner.

These are the simple rewards that can be given out daily, the nuances in their lifts, the adjustments to their movements, the weight they were able to handle. All these little victories should be pointed out as they happen. People need verbal rewards more than material rewards in the gym. They will reward themselves with the way their clothes fit and the comments they'll acquire.

CHAPTER 10
HATE THE TRAINER/
LOVE THE TRAINER

"I'm all out of nice..."

It's not easy to be the person everyone loves to hate. As a trainer, you become more critical than an architect and more informed than a hairdresser. You see beautiful women at their worst - no makeup, sweating, panting, reddened, complaining, hungover, garlic-breathed, sleep-deprived, unshaven legs and ripped shorts with pulled back hair and an evil eye usually reserved for loved ones - and yet, you still see their beauty.

You have men who complain about work, co-workers, traffic, any type of roadblocks in their lives from their spouse to their kids to their sex lives. There really is no sacred ground and you are the path of least resistance. You are the captive audience. Get used to it, but let it all roll off your back.

You are the necessary evil in their lives. To some, you are the reason they get up in the morning. Rarely do you see the fruits of your labor. You don't get invited to their parties, don't see them in real clothes, don't get introduced respectfully in public, if at all, and yet, you are their most valuable asset.

They call you at dinner and before lunch for advice on the menu, yet, would never invite you to lunch They don't appreciate you enough for one second to say thank you when you affirm, positively, that they're improving. Yet you keep telling them.

They loudly say they hate you, call you a jerk, a loser, insane - yes, sometimes even spit on you or in your direction. You show up daily, weekly, hourly, nodding in agreement as they bitch about their pillows not being fluffed high enough. You smile and laugh with undivided attention, despite the flat tire you may have had on the way over, or the fact that your heart aches for your kid whom you only saw for 10 minutes, before having to run to the gym.

It's a thankless job, yet worth every drop of sweat. You're a counselor, psychiatrist, motivator, comforter, negotiator, dream interpreter, dietician, dog trainer and friend. Their health is your mission; their future's, in your hands. Their weaknesses, your blame. Their metamorphosis, their own.

The tropical vacation they're so intently focused on with heart, mind and body, will never be your own. All the strength you use each day to meet them, comes only from the belief in yourself to say you can, and they can. It's a mutual admiration club, but they don't know "you're President."

KICK THEM OUT OF THE NEST

As a trainer you must understand that people are not something you can put on cruise control. They need your attention, encouragement, opinions and direction. They need validation and motivation and sometimes just a place to vent.

You must not take any of it personally. You must be a looking glass that only reflects back their best aspects. Remain objective, calm, level and attentive. Be honest, but know where to draw the line before hurting them.

They don't have to and often don't, show gratitude. Sometimes you'll feel invisible. Do what you are paid to do and then a little extra, and you will always be working. Most of all, teach them enough to set them free, with knowledge, confidence and understanding of what they asked to learn from you.

Genuinely care for them, for they are your co-worker. If you're being paid to do something, you'd better do it!! But never the bare minimum, always go further. Always offer more. But never cross the line between professionalism and friendship. You can be friendly, be amicable, and be their confidante, but keep it in the gym.

BE STRICT

There are many times when the client would rather talk than work out. You must rein them in and keep them moving. They will have excuses and distractions and do everything they can to slow down the workout.

You must be strict in keeping the pace because you understand something they don't; pace is a big part of the pump, and of the development of the whole muscle system in responding to breath, movement, strength, stamina and endurance.

They wouldn't train for a marathon by running in one minute increments. Don't let them train for shape by long pauses that cut the effectiveness of the workout in half. Don't let them state the rate of work by inordinate pauses and conversations. Keep them moving.

BE CONSISTENT

Be consistent in how you run the program as well. Keep their concentration level on the movements and not on trivial stories about your workout history or weekend antics. If you have something to offer about your particular approach to a particular movement - a feeling, a result, a stance or vision - use it to enhance their particular experience in the given movement.

If your plan is to work certain bodyparts on certain days, or certain exercises, sets or rep schemes, stay true to them so they can measure their own progress. It's good to add a surprise every once in a while, but stay consistent more of the time.

There is a reason professional teams, high school teams, the military and every level of conditioning that has to do with physical work, has a certain daily discipline they follow, first thing. Obviously, it builds character; but it also starts a natural rhythm into their lives that makes stretching and warm-ups as much a part of their day as eating, sleeping, brushing their teeth.

You help build this consistency by going through a series of exercises that encourage the capability of the client, workout to workout; and make it simple enough to have them perform it on their own. Get them to this point of doing it themselves, where they look forward to it, where they'll begin on their own if you're not there for their arrival.

Consistency has to be attended to across the board, training, eating, sleeping, recuperating, supplementing; only then will you be able to recognize any flaws that may be leading to less than optimal conditioning. If the client falls short in any of these areas, it is up to you to correct and encourage filling the gaps. If you at least acknowledge areas that are lacking, you will not be responsible for what the client is doing in their off time. Remember, you only get them a few hours per week, you do your best at that time, but make them accountable for their free time as well.

CHAPTER 11

11 TIPS TO BE A BETTER TRAINER

1. When a new customer comes to the counter, they are your responsibility. They need to be greeted with a handshake, a water, a towel, a smile, something to greet them and let them know you are happy to have them as a guest in your "house."

2. Do not sit at the counter when a guest walks in. Let me repeat again - greet them at your door, from a standing position, eye to eye, with a smile and a "hello."

3. A trainer cannot expect to tutor a client if they're unwilling to even give them directions to the locker room? If they mumble through their protocol, how on earth can they ever convince a customer to enlist them for an hour of tuition when they can't understand them for one minute? Stand up and talk!

4. They are there to put their trust in you. They expect you to give them honest information, insights, and safe methods for achieving their goals. The quicker you can establish their trust, by enlisting yourself in their welfare, the deeper the tie and the easier the sale.

5. Training is about trust. It's about relationships. It's about keeping them on task because they've already proven to themselves that they can't or don't want to do it alone. That's why they came to you.

6. You must proceed with the endgoal in mind. You must see what they cannot. You must draw "a picture of

possibility." And you must ultimately believe in it as much or more than them.

7.   Paste emotion to that picture - how they will feel, the comments they'll look forward to, the way clothes will feel and fit - and the work for both of you will come that much easier.

8. Now, paste a loved one into their picture. How would their spouse respond to their improved fitness? How would it help influence their sons, daughters and family members? What kind of example would they bring to their coworkers, associates and friends? The ripple effect they cannot perceive is something you already know as fact. Sell it. Convince.

9. Assure them that almost everyone is a beginner, everyone has their own interests at heart, and are not concerned with how you look, what you wear, or what you lift.

10. ASK YOURSELF: What is my sales pitch? What am I saying to the potential client? How accountable am I to them? Are you serious enough to enlist your time and effort into achieving their needs? Are you doing it for the money? You either have integrity or have deceit.

11. ASK THEM: How serious are YOU about getting in shape? How much time will YOU invest in YOUR goals? Do YOU understand that it takes more than an hour workout commitment to achieve results? Where do YOU want to be in 1, 3, 6 months? Do YOU have limitations? Injuries? Priorities? Sports YOU participate in? TALK TO THEM ABOUT THEM.

MORE BOOKS BY THE AUTHOR
"SST SIMPLE STRUCTURED TRAINING"
How The Mind Trains The Body

"SHOCK AND AWE MUSCLE"
Stage Ready Definition That Shocks And Awes Mere Mortals

Both available on the Kindle Platform and _amazon.com_

You can also email _tom@TomTypinski.com_
Please feel free to ask questions about training, workouts, competitive physique and corporate wellness engagements.

View his Facebook sites: Dream Video Bikini, Bodybuilding, Figure & Fitness Fans
ShockAndAweMuscle.com
Twitter: @TomTypinski
and YouTube/TomTypinski

www.ingramcontent.com/pod-product-compliance
Lightning Source LLC
Chambersburg PA
CBHW022135280326
41933CB00007B/699